101 Ways to Lose Your Belly Fat

By Laura Pierce

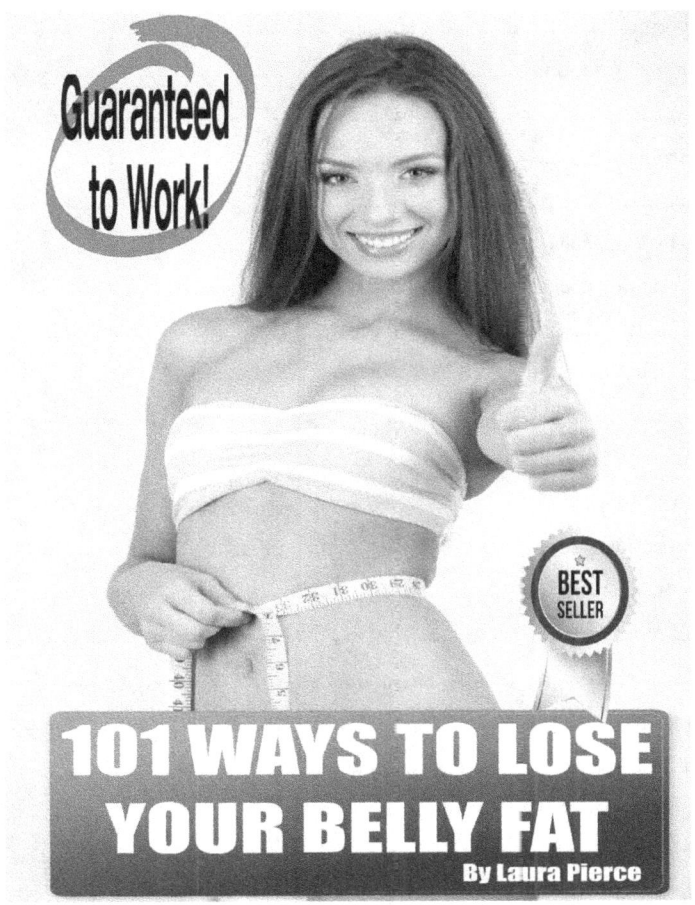

101 Ways to Lose Your Belly Fat

By Laura Pierce

Contents

101 Ways to Lose Your Belly Fat

By Laura Pierce

101 Ways to Lose Your Belly Fat

By Laura Pierce

101 Ways to Lose Your Belly Fat

By Laura Pierce

101 Ways to Lose Your Belly Fat

By Laura Pierce

101 Tips for Successful Dieting

1. Starting a diet program.
Dieting, just like any other plan that requires discipline and commitment such as fitness, can only succeed if you don't lose sight of your set goals. First, you need to determine if you are ready to go all the way to achieve your objectives without getting sidetracked.

2. Acceptance and taking action.
Most people find it easy to live in denial since they won't have to face the harsh realities of their situation. Being overweight is not the end of life and accepting that you have a problem is actually the first step towards a healthy and beautiful you. You stand a better chance of attaining your dieting goals if you tackle your weight problems head on and as soon as possible. Remember, excuses and denial won't change a thing but, instead reduce your chances of ever turning your life around.

3. Fact finding.
Information is power and you can't do much if don't know exactly what you are doing. Gather and analyze information from different sources to be in the loop about the latest dieting practices, nutritional facts on different types of foods and special recipes. Please CLICK HERE for some great dieting tips and food recipes.

4. Focus and determination.

Find a way to constantly remind yourself of why you need a diet plan in the first place so as not to lose focus on your goals. There are all sorts of reasons why people diet, for instance improved physical appearance, health, or just to look like beauty models. Whatever your reasons for dieting may be, you need to stay on track and relentlessly pursue your objectives.

5. Make it personal.

Making your dieting plan personal is an excellent way to jump start it. This is simply because you'll always be able to fuel the desire, stirring inside you in order to achieve your fitness goals and keep yourself on the success trajectory. Routine things like taking your weight, trying new outfits and comparing your image to photos of yester years, can go a long way to helping you keep the dieting fire burning. Emotions play a major in motivation and you seeing positive changes in your posture, physical appearance or weight could be just the thing you need to help you stay on track.

6. Yes, you can diet successfully.

Stop viewing dieting as an impossible feat instead, remind yourself of what have or can achieve if you stick to the diet plan. Your mind can play tricks on you by making a mole hill appear as a big mountain, so fill our thoughts with positive images that will see you desire to attain our goals. Remember, it takes time to see tangible results and don't be in hurry to transform overnight since you risk harming yourself in the process.

7. Choose the right dieting program.

You should not just embark on any dieting program before considering the pros and cons. In fact, you should evaluate the different types of diet programs out there to identify the most suitable for you because you can't succeed in something that you don't have confidence in pursuing. Review feedback from friends, colleagues or relatives who have gone through dieting to help you identify a good program.

8. Positive images.

Staying on a diet can be a daunting task without positive imagery and affirmations to reassure yourself. Our actions are greatly influenced by what we think or believe and you don't want to fill your mind with negative thoughts that will only derail your dieting program. A positive mindset will help you start dieting and see it through to completion.

9. You can't stand alone.

Support and encouragement from close friends and family can come in handy in moments when you are about to throw in the towel. While family and friends are commonly known to be a constant source of ridicule, they can also be a source of strength and inspiration in your lowest moments once they come to appreciate how committed you are in your dieting program.

10. Dieting the fun way.

Dieting can be pure hell, if your kitchen is stocked with the very types of food that you are trying to avoid or if our diet is composed only of the types of food that are not appealing. You can make your life a little easier by starting with healthy food that are also palatable. In addition, try to stock your refrigerator with only the healthy foods in your diet plan.

11. Eat only when hungry.

Make sure that you only eat to satisfy hunger because other factors such as stress, addiction, etc. can also make you crave for food when you actually don't need it. It's always important to determine why you feel like eating something and only eat when you are really hungry. Alternatively, you can just drink water if unsure or munch on a healthy snack.

12. Avoid foods with MSG.

Foods containing MSG do more harm than good to your body and should be avoided at all costs. Lots of foods out there are nowadays infused with MSG, especially the highly processed foods. Such foods have little or none nutritional value and will instead deposit more fat into your body. You will do yourself more good by avoiding such foods with MSG.

13. Get adequate rest and sleep.

It's important for the body to get enough sleep so as to rejuvenate, clear toxins and to repair damaged tissues. Lack of enough sleep has a detrimental effect on the body because as the body tries to compensate for lack of sleep, the rate of food metabolism is reduced and the appetite is heightened –a perfect recipe for weight increase.

14. Incorporate fiber rich foods.

Your diet is not complete without fiber. Fiber benefits the body in so many ways, such as flushing out toxins, reducing food cravings, promoting complete digestion and lowering up build of cholesterol in the blood. For more information about the benefits of fiber in your diet, please read this book The Fat Loss Factor.

15. Customize your diet program.

In as much as there are many diet programs out there that you can follow, you stand to benefit more if your chosen program is personalized around your own unique lifestyle and needs. Work with a qualified nutritionist to help you design a custom diet program for your unique needs.

16. Mind your calorie intake.

You cannot achieve your dieting goals using guess work. You need to determine the amount of calories contained in the foods that you eat, how much calories your body burns and your day to day tasks since you can reduce weight by consuming less calories, and metabolizing more. Pay more attention to the nutritional information of foods to determine their caloric content.

17. Avoid soft drinks.

Soft drinks such as Sodas are fortified with high calories that can only accelerate your weight gain. You can instead drink fresh fruit juices or pure water, which is not adulterated with dangerous chemicals and calories. Even diet sodas still have trace amounts of additives and calories

18. Eat only to get nutrients.

Do not overindulge in food but eat to provide your body with the necessary nutrients to support healthy living. Some people eat as a way of coping with stressful situations or to satisfy a craving to their own endangerment. People gain weight because of excess food which are converted to fat and consequently deposited into the body.

19. Avoid junk foods.

Junk foods are highly processed and thus mostly filled with fats and cholesterol. But, with more and more fast food chains springing up at almost every corner, most people find themselves visiting these joints which hardly serve wholesome meals. You may have to carry a lunch box to the office next time in order to stay on track of your diet program.

20. Eat low caloric and harder to metabolize foods.

Eat foods such as apples, celery and vegetables that have low calories and are harder to metabolize to intake low amounts calories because your body will need to use more energy to burn them. In addition, you'll be consuming fewer calories –thus facilitating your weight loss program.

21. Eat at a slower rate.

When you eat slowly, you would be able to consume the amount of calories that your body needs to function properly without going overboard. This happens because it takes a specific duration of time for your stomach to signal your brain that you have taken the required amount of food. But, when you eat fast, you are likely to consume more food than what you actually need.

22. Healthy breakfast.

Make sure your breakfast consists of proteins, fruits, and foods rich in healthy fats for example eggs and bacon. Traditional breakfast meals are mostly made up of cereals such as doughnuts, bagels, etc. These types of food contain high sugar levels and can exponentially increase your insulin levels. Make sure your breakfast meal is not 100% carbs for a healthy diet.

23. Don't drink while eating

Did you know drinking a lot of fluids during meals can lead to binge eating? It's not advisable to intake lots of drinks during meals as this can make your stomach bloated. In fact, nutritionists recommend that you should take a drink (preferably a glass of water) only after 10-15 minutes of having meals.

24. Always chew food thoroughly.

Always chew your food thoroughly when eating to ensure proper digestion and metabolism. In addition, thorough chewing also promotes eating food at the right speed. Take your time to savor and chew your food to facilitate digestion and assimilation.

25. Don't eat prior to going to sleep.

It's advisable to take your supper at least 3 hours before going to bed to prevent accumulation of excess sugars which are consequently converted to fats. When you fall asleep, your body's metabolism rate slows down would not be able to digest all the food but, instead accumulate the excess calories.

26. Get rid of all unhealthy foods.

Prevention is better than cure. Thus, your life will be a lot easier if you're not bombarded with tempting food at every nook and cranny of your house. Clear your kitchen of all unhealthy foodstuffs and replace them with healthy foods recommended in your diet program.

27. Choose whey protein drinks.

If your diet entails drinking protein drinks to boost protein levels in your body, you should go with whey protein drinks instead of soy protein. This is mainly because whey protein is easily absorbed by the body and also does not have harmful side effects on your body.

28. Increase intake of spicy foods.

Eating spicy foods normally cause people to sweat exceedingly. This is because the spices accelerate the body's metabolism rate causing you to perspire. Spices help your body to burn more calories, especially fats, facilitating your weight reduction program. Therefore, don't hold back next time you spice your food with chilies —it does not only make your food taste better but, also helps you lose weight.

29. Eat more fruits and vegetables.

Fruits and vegetables are rich in vitamins such as Vitamins A, B and C as well as minerals and enzymes. However, you can only unlock their full potential if taken in their uncooked state. Heat can easily destroy many essential nutrients found in vegetables and fruits. This is why over cooked or processed foods are not recommended for those on a diet.

30. Go for healthier snacks.

Snacks may come in handy when you want something to munch to pass time or to satisfy a craving. However, to ensure that you don't gain extra weight, only consume healthier foods such as fruits, nuts, vegetables, yoghurt etc. to ensure that your body is not overloaded with non-essential calories.

31. Organic food is healthy.

While the benefits of fruits and vegetables may be apparent to everyone, not every fresh food is healthy. You need to be more careful when shopping for food and avoid non-organic foods that are grown using fertilizers and harmful chemicals. The foods that are not grown organically can expose you to various unwarranted side effects and sicknesses.

32. Avoid simple sugars.

Simple carbs have high glycemic content and should be avoided at all costs since they can your blood cholesterol to dangerous levels. You'll do yourself a lot of good by eating foods composed of complex carbohydrates which are harder to metabolize. This prevents you from consuming excess calories and at the same time promoting complete digestion.

33. Only eat at the dining table.

It's easier to lose track of your calorie intake if you have the tendency to eat everywhere and at any time since you can go easily overindulge without realizing it. If your goal is to lose weight, then you should restrict eating to your dining table and at specified times. Eating while doing activities such as watching a movie or playing computer games can interfere with your brain's ability to determine whether you have had enough food.

34. Eat before shopping for grocery.

When you go shopping for grocery on an empty stomach you can find yourself buying or even munching on foods that are not listed on your shopping list. The temptation to buy unhealthy foods can be so great that you can totally disregard your diet program. Play it safe by eating something before you go to the grocery store.

This way, you can have better control on what to buy and to stick to your diet plan.

35. Avoid restaurant foods.

Most meals served in restaurants are not healthy because they cooked with a lot of oil and are also highly processed. Dieting can be a daunting task in an environment full of tempting food that you are not supposed to eat. Eating out does more harm than good because you'll always be tempted to divert from your dieting program by the sweet aroma of unhealthy foods wafting to your nostrils.

36. Avoid situations that can trigger food cravings.

Certain factors such as stress, loneliness, and conflicts can trigger a strong desire to eat food at moments when you don't really have to eat. You need to determine what makes you crave for food and find alternative ways to cope nstead of indulging in eating or snacking.

37. Keep track of your progress.

When dieting, especially to lose weight, you need to measure, record and evaluate your performance over a specific period of time. This way, you'll be able to visualize your progress and to determine where to make adjustments so as to stay on track of your diet program. If your goal is to lose weight, weigh yourself periodically to find out if your dieting effort is paying off. Plus, seeing a record of our performance can in fact help boost your morale to continue with dieting.

38. Limit your food intake.

Exercise control over your food portions to ensure you don't overeat. Eat from a smaller plate to make sure you don't serve more food than you are supposed to since you won't be able to serve more food than the plate can accommodate.

39. Eat wholesome meals.

Ensure that your body gets all the required nutrients at every meal time. Make it a routine to incorporate different types of food, including fruits, vegetables and fiber to reduce craving for the types of food that your body lacks. A balanced diet can help keep your appetite in check.

40. Savor your meals.

Take your time to appreciate food using your sense of smell, taste, sight and texture. Eating food should not be a tasking obligation but, an all inclusive and pleasant experience touching on all your five senses. Savoring food also makes you eat slowly, thereby facilitating your weight loss program. Please read my book Fat Loss Factor to learn some great recipes to try on your own.

41. Cut down on chocolates.

A lot of people, mainly women find it irresistible to eat chocolates. However, if you wish to accomplish your fitness goals, then you should cut down your cravings for their sweet taste. Just keep in mind that chocolates are filled with high quantities of fats and energy, which is capable of making you, put on more weight. Therefore, you must not incorporate them into your shopping list.

42. Observe your BMI.

Be extra familiar with your Basal Metabolic Rate. The Basal Metabolic Rate is the best method to measure wellbeing and weight loss progress. The Body Mass Index (BMI) is just the measurement of your height to weight ratio and will not take into account your muscle mass.

43. Reward your dieting efforts more often.

Whenever you achieve your diet goals, for instance, when you lose 5-10 pounds in a given period of dieting, you need to devise creative ways to motivate yourself. For example, you can buy small sized clothes that you keep on trying. This way, you'll be able to rekindle your desire to attain your fitness goals.

44. Acquire a diet plan journal.

Use a dieting chronicle or any other notebook to keep a record of the foods that you eat on a daily basis. Apart from that, the record book should also include the types of food you are planning on eating for the subsequent days. This way, you can prevent unplanned meals, and be on your way to success with your diet program.

45. Be more active around the house.

While dieting, you stand to gain more if you avoid things that can make you store extra fats for instance, sitting idly on the sofa or just lazing around the house. Increase your daily duties and avoid things like watching the TV the whole day while munching on snacks. Engaging in physical activities by doing routine tasks in the house can also help you burn those extra calories.

46. Exercise your mind while riding a train or bus.

Whether you are using a bus or train to go to work, there are many ways that you can exercise your mind and burn excess calories. One technique is to answer a crossword puzzle, Sudoku or to play any type of mind boggling games that requires reasoning and strategy. This would improve your brain power, and at the same time facilitates your weight loss program by burning up even more calories.

47. Use smaller eating utensils.

If the main objective of your diet program is weight loss, then you need to control your food intake. This is the time to purchase smaller dining and kitchen utensils. Having small size eating utensils, would ensure that you serve smaller amounts of food. In addition, it would also help you limit your serving portions.

48. Join an online diet community.

There are a number of people out there who are involved in various types of weight loss programs. To reach out to them, the only thing that you need to do is to register with any of the online weight loss diet forums. Once you are a signed up, you can engage with other members, share your dieting experience and also learn from their experiences. Apart from that, you'll also get more motivated to achieve your goals seeing that you are not alone.

49. Monitor your progress with a weighing scale.

To properly monitor your advancement through your selected diet program, it is best if you use a scale for it. However, you should not use it excessively. If you step on the weighing machine every day, you actually wouldn't be able to be conscious of your weight loss. Preferably, you should do it at least once weekly, so that you can see a significant difference. You also need to realize that weight loss isn't the only factor that is of major concern. In this book Fat Loss Factor, we are going to discover several novel techniques that you can use to accurately measure key milestones in your diet program.

50. Stay away from coffee shops.

When you are on a diet program, it can be a great idea to stay away from your favorite coffee joint. Since, most of the time, when you walk into a coffee shop, you may end up buying not just a cup of coffee, but in addition one or two of their scrumptious pastries. Apart from that, iced coffees can also be loaded with extra calories that your body doesn't want.

51. The power of positive thinking.

Thinking positive is not just about personal development programs. But, can also be used to help you burn calories through a suitable diet program. For example, if you have not made up your mind on how long you want to follow a diet plan, then filling your mind with positive thoughts could help relieve any anxiety. When you talk yourself into believing that you can do it through the power of positive thinking, you will eventually have the drive to keep up with your diet plan and to accomplish your dreams.

52. Reduce the intervals between your main meals.

You should not take more than 3 hours before eating something. Since, when you stay for too long between meals or snacking, it can in fact lead to binge eating. Therefore, you should make it a habit to munch on something healthy, at least every 2-3 hours.

53. Be aware of the dangers of obesity.

Write down all the disadvantages and dangers of being overweight. When your listing is done, put it on the door of your refrigerator. This way, you will always be reminded of the penalty of over eating unhealthy foods, every time you open your refrigerator door. This will help you not to lose focus on your goals to consistently follow your diet plan.

54. Incorporate foods rich in protein in all meals.

Each time you have a meal, you are supposed to include foods containing protein, for example eggs, fish, chicken, lean meat etc. By doing that, you can make certain that you are supplying your body with more bodybuilding nutrients. Apart, from that, you will also be suppressing your appetite, because proteins are typically harder to digest.

55. Stick to your home cooked food, even at the office.

Once you go to work, you may be tempted to pay a quick visit to the fast food chain in the neighborhood to have lunch. Since eating at a fast food restaurant may encourage you to have unhealthy meals, then it's best to carry your own home cooked meal. This way, you won't only be ensuring that you stick to your diet plan, but it can as well help you cut down your expenses.

56. Include eggs in your breakfast.

When you do breakfast, it's best if you include eggs in it.
This is because eggs are packed with an important protein called albumin. Apart from that, it can also provide you with energy giving nutrients. Hence, it can help you attain higher metabolism rates, and would also provide you with more energy throughout the day. For a great breakfast recipes, read my book here.

57. Avoid beer.

If you normally drink beers on your own or with friends, then you may have to cut down your intake. Since, beers are loaded with plenty of calories. For that reason, it is not a good idea to drink too much, especially if you are on a diet, since it may avert you from achieving your goals.

58. Choose a diet program that works for you.

Keep in mind that not all diet programs can work for everyone. For that reason, you should only follow a program, which you believe works for you. This way, you won't have to force yourself into doing things that you don't want. Apart from that, this can also make your desired goals more achievable.

59. Acquire a passionate aspiration to lose weight.

When you have a strong desire to lose weight, then each time you wake up in the morning, you'd already be thinking about how to accomplish it. Thus, it is better if you think of various ways that can make you really lose weight. One way to achieve this is to visualize yourself looking fit whenever you look at yourself in the mirror. Aside from that, you can also boost up your morale by trying smaller sized clothes to see if they can fit.

60. Set short term and attainable goals to achieve the long term goals.

If your main objective is to lose fifteen pounds in 6 weeks or more but, you see it as an impossible task, then you should consider setting short term goals for it. With that illustration, you can actually begin with a goal of losing about 1 pound per week, which is more attainable. Since short term goals are easier to accomplish, you must focus more on it, so that you can ultimately attain the other one. In my diet plan, we create a specific target setting worksheet to make it easier for you to accomplish your goals. **Check it out here.**

61. Take snapshots of yourself.

Before beginning your weight loss program, you should take a snapshot of yourself. This way, you would have a record that you can judge against, after several weeks of dieting. This will help motivate you more, and ensure that you remain consistent.

62. Aim to look like a model.

There are specific Television channels that showcase models adorning the newest fashion styles. Since these models look athletic, you would be more motivated to put in more effort on your own diet program, so as to attain an awesome figure just like them. Do it more often, so that you don't forget your target in achieving your dreams.

63. Focus on building more muscles while dieting.

If you want to get a model's physique, which could be the main reason you are on a diet, you should also exercise to build additional muscle mass. This is because muscles need more calories to maintain. In other words, the more muscles you are able to build, the more calories your body would burn, which results in losing weight.

64. Find a reliable partner.

Dieting can actually be fun; if you workout with one partner or partners. You can also do it with a relative or a close friend. In doing so, all of you would be in a position to assist one another with moral support and solidarity. Apart from that, you can also share your progress more often and to keep each other from losing focus.

65. Foster the spirit of competition.

In case you can get hold of someone whom you can go through the weight loss program together, then you should make it a contest. That way, you can both compare your weight lose progress side by side and week by week. Apart from that, you can also set a certain target, and provide a reward to the winner who has attained it.

66. Contemplate on your set goals before sleeping.

Whenever you lie down to sleep on your bed, try to visualize how great you would feel and look like, once you have lost a considerable amount of body weight. This way, you would become more excited to doing the things you need in order to achieve your dreams. Thus, you would be motivated to continue eating healthier types of foods, and getting sufficient exercise.

67. Think twice, before eating an unhealthy food.

Anytime you are about to eat junk foodstuff, chocolate, sweets or ice cream, you ought to think first. You should seriously consider whether consuming an unhealthy foodstuff would be worth the consequences, the troubles that you have gone through to lose weight. Doing this may actually help you stop craving for dangerous foodstuffs, and instead prefer healthier foods.

68. Drink pure water.

Anytime you are feeling thirsty, you should drink a cold glass of water. Cold water can help your body burn calories faster. This way, you would be able to lose more fats and calories and eventually lose weight. Hence, you should prepare some ice cubes or place some water in a container and put in your refrigerator to cool down.

69. Selective snacking.
One of the most dangerous practices that can make you lose sight of your goals is eating snack items that are not healthy, especially before going to bed. Thus, if you merely need to eat before going to sleep, in that case you should choose something that won't give you too much calories. A good example would be a packet of cookies that only contains a few hundred calories.

70. Reward yourself with your favorite foods.
Even whilst you are on a diet, you can occasionally enjoy favorite foods. However, you should do it in moderation. When you have a meal of your favorite foods, you wouldn't feel that your diet is too grueling to keep up with. For this reason, you would be motivated to follow it through to the end.

71. Use cinnamon on your yoghurt.
Eating yoghurt is actually one of the best ways to lose extra weight. However, to make it taste better, you can sprinkle cinnamon on it. Doing so would not just improve the taste of yoghurt. Yoghurt can actually boost your metabolism and help burn additional calories.

72. Drink carrot juice.
When you are thirsty and craving for a different drink other than water, then you should go for a glass of carrot juice as an alternative. Carrot juice is packed with fiber, which can help you

not just to metabolize fats, but also to suppress your desire for food. Therefore, you ought to ensure it is a regular item to accompany your diet.

73. Calcium supplement.

Partaking calcium supplements regularly can actually help you lose more fats. Because it makes you full of energy. Calcium plus phosphorus and Vitamin D3 can really increase your calorie levels, and as a result enable you to perform more strenuous activities day in day out.

74. Learn how to handle stress in the workplace.

Stress is one of the factors that can cause many people to overeat in eating especially at work. Thus, it is very important if you are familiar with techniques of managing stress. One proven technique that can help calm you down is to practice deep breathing in and out, at any time you feel stressed at work or at home. This can make it easier for you to calm down, control your temper and avoid food cravings.

75. Eat a banana every morning.

Every time you get up in the morning, munch on a banana and wash it down with a full glass of water. This will provide you with the calories that your body requires to face the day. In addition, banana also helps in keeping your appetite in check for the rest of the day.

76. Eating healthy snacks.

Anytime you munch on something between main meals, you should ensure that the snack you eat is healthy as well. A good example of a nutritious snack would be a piece of chicken breast.

Given that chicken is an excellent source of protein, it can assist your body in building additional muscle tissues. Apart from that, protein is in reality harder to digest, which is a good thing since it can help you control the size your portion when serving meals.

77. Apply soy sauce to suppress hunger.
Taking soy sauce with your meals can actually do you more good than just improving the taste of your food. With respect to the latest research findings, soy proteins found in soy sauce can network with your brain receptors. Their networking with the brain neurons can result in making you feel satisfied quicker than usual.

78. Eat eggs with watermelon.
If you want a great breakfast recipe for your weight loss plan, then you should try eating watermelon and eggs for breakfast. It is even better if you take the melon first, followed by the eggs. Melons are overflowing with vitamins, as well as water and fiber, which can make you the feel satisfied faster. When you later eat eggs, it will help break down the carbs in the melon, in addition to providing you with essential proteins.

79. Partake a glass of wine daily.
Drinking even one glass of wine every day, preferably during dinner, can facilitate you in attaining your fitness goals. This is so because wine contains Resveratrol from the grapefruit, which prevents the growth of fat cells, particularly in the region of your belly. Apart from that, it can also significantly boost your body's metabolism rate.

80. Incorporate pomegranates in your diet plan.

There is a popular misconception that eating this fruit can even make you put on weight, for the reason of its taste. On the contrary, in spite of being so sweet, eating this fruit can actually help you in suppressing your appetite for sweet snacks. Apart from that, the seeds of this fruit can lower the capability of your body to store fats.

81. Eating barbequed meat.

If you like eating meat, especially during weekends, you should eat even more barbeque. Whenever you barbeque meat, you are actually burning up more of its fat, in the process of cooking it. As a result, it is now time to fire up that barbecue grill, so that you continue to enjoy your meat without having to be concerned about getting fat.

82. Eat more spinach.

Next time you go shopping for green vegetables at the grocery store, you should make spinach your priority more than the other types of greens. This is simply because spinach contains more fiber than the other types of vegetables. Eating more food rich in fiber, would help your body to burn more fats, as well as suppressing your appetite.

83. Eat only healthy cheese.

If you are the kind of person who loves cheese, as an alternative to the regular cheese, you should purchase the one made from goat's milk. Since cheese products prepared from goat's milk are essentially lower in calories, than those made from the cow's milk by about 40%. Thus, you should try to use this type of cheese if you want to lose weight.

84. Eat more of good fats to do away with bad fats.

Eating the healthy type of fats is one of the proven ways to do away with the bad fats. Some of the best sources of healthy fats include rapeseed oil, walnuts, and eggs. Apart from helping your body in burning up excess fats, they can also reduce your risk to contract heart diseases.

85. Include oats in your breakfast.

Many people nowadays eat cooked oats for breakfast in order to lose weight. Well, this can in fact help you lose weight because oats are packed with lots of fiber. When you eat a breakfast that is loaded with fiber, it would cause you to feel full even when it is almost lunch time. As a consequence, it can help you be in charge of your servings during meals.

86. Eating an apple before meals.

Eating at least one apple per day would not just prevent disease, but can also rid your body of fats and harmful toxins. Simply eat an apple about 20 minutes before eating food. This can effectively help to suppress your desire to eat more food and consequently help you consume lesser amounts of food.

87. Use olive oil.

Eating salads is safe as long as you regulate the quantities that you consume. Thus, you can only keep from gaining weight if you take charge of your salad servings. Another thing to do to help you enjoy your salad without worrying about weight gain is to take a salad with olive oil; olive oil has healthy fatty acids that also help in suppressing your appetite.

88. Eat more often.

Contrary to popular beliefs, eating more in a day can actually help you cut down weight. All you have to do is pay close attention to the quantities that you eat so that you don't overindulge. Eat at least 6 times in a day instead of usual 3 times per day. Munching on something between the main meals can enhance your metabolism rate because your body would be constantly burning the foods that you consume.

89. Top up your sandwiches with tomato slices.

Whenever you eat a sandwich, either for breakfast or as a snack, try to top it up with tomatoes. This would help make you satisfied longer. In addition, tomatoes also contain enzymes, which can help inhibit the release of the hormone known as ghrelin. This is the hormone that is responsible for controlling hunger pangs.

90. Eat pineapples.

Pineapple fruit is one of the best foods to eat if you are on a weight loss program. This is mainly because; it contains bromolina which makes it easier for the body to break down proteins. It also has large quantities of fiber and can effectively boost your metabolism rate, especially when eaten as a snack.

91. Eat more oranges.

Oranges also can help you lose more weight, because it contains elevated levels of Vitamin C. Vitamin C is essentially one of the best substances, which can effectively convert fats into energy. Thus, every time you eat oranges, know that you are actually aiding your body to burn your excess fats to produce energy. On top of that, oranges are also good sources of fiber, which helps in suppressing food cravings.

92. Share your meals with a friend.
Various studies show that people who invite their friends over for meals tend to eat the same amounts of food as their guests. Therefore, you should eat more with friends who are also on diet, or those who don't consume too much food. For instance, if you are a man, then eat with a lady friend since women often eat less food than men. This way, you will be able to eat smaller quantities of food than when you are eating alone.

93. Avoid energy drinks.
Even though some people believe that drinking energy drinks only boosts energy levels, they actually cause more harm than good for someone on a weight loss program. This happens because energy drinks, deliver their energy too quickly such that your body won't be able to burn them but, instead convert the excess energy into fats.

94. Drink skimmed milk instead of regular milk.
In as much as drinking milk is not good for your body since it has very high fat content, you can still take milk without compromising your health by switching to skimmed milk. However, should avoid milk altogether to prevent adding excess body fat and inflammations. Other safe alternatives include almond and coconut milk which do not put your health at risk.

95. Use Apple Cider vinegar on your sauces and puddings.

Sauces and salads that include apple cider vinegar can really make it easier for your body to burn more fats. Since Apple Cider contains acetic acid, which can enhance your body's ability to burn calories and fats.

96. Choose a suitable diet program.

Your diet can go totally wrong if it is not compatible with your unique situation. Therefore, to choose a suitable diet plan, it is best not to go to consider various options out there. Just make sure that your selected plan is not too constraining. Since, a wrong program can make your body go on a defensive mode and consequently setting a chain of events to counter react to your diet program. Fat Loss Factor is a flexible program that is simple and can be personalized to suit your lifestyle.

97. Visit the toilet at least twice per day.

If you get at least two bowel movements per day, you would be more conscious of the foods that you eat. Apart from that, you'll also become extra vigilant on the quantity of water that you drink each day. All in all, having more bowel movements will help you observe a healthy diet plan.

98. Drink fresh fruit juice.

Drinking freshly squeezed fruit juice made from real fruits is by far the best way to drink juice as opposed to the flavored juices made from synthetic chemicals and food color. Fresh fruit juices are filled with vitamins and minerals that can help your body to remain healthy. In addition, fruit juices also contain nutrients that suppress appetite, making you feel satisfied for a longer time.

99. Take green tea to burn more fats.

Drinking green tea can also help you cut down weight, in addition to your diet plan because it burns fat very fast. Aside from that, green tea can also increase your energy reserves to enable you perform more physical duties. Plus, it also boosts the immune system.

100. Set realistic goals.

You should not have unrealistic expectations before starting a weight loss program. Since, you can easily get discouraged before attaining any concrete goals. Therefore, you should set goals that are achievable, so that you can maintain with your diet program consistently without losing focus of your set goals until you attain them.

101. Determine the correct portion sizes.

Determining the accurate portion sizes is one the most contentious issues in dieting. In spite of the thousands of bits of information available out there, many people are still confused about the right quantity of food that they should eat when dieting. Nevertheless, if you are not sure, you can use your fist as a standard such that whenever you serve food, you make sure that it does not exceed the size of your fist. Well, thanks for reading up to this point; I hope you have found this information helpful! Anyways, click here for more tips on dieting and some healthy food recipes.